Easy Vegan Air Fryer Recipes for Beginners

Cheap Delicacies for your Everyday Dishes

Samantha Attanasio

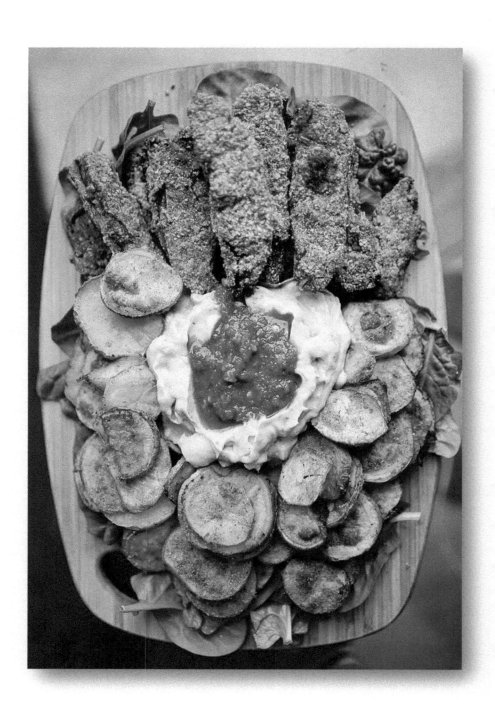

by reading this document, the reader agrees that under no circumstances is the author responsible for any losses, direct or indirect, which are incurred as a result of the use of information contained within this document, including, but not limited to, — errors, omissions, or inaccuracies.

Table of Contents

Vegetable

Ratatouille

Preparation time: 20 minutes

Cooking time: 25 minutes

Servings: 4

Ingredients:

- One sprig basil
- One sprig flat-leaf parsley
- One sprig mint
- One tbsp. coriander powder
- One tsp. capers
- ½ lemon, juiced
- Salt and ground black pepper, to taste
- Two eggplants sliced crosswise
- Two red onions, chopped
- Four cloves garlic, minced
- Two red peppers sliced crosswise
- One fennel bulb cut crosswise
- Three large zucchinis sliced crosswise
- Five tbsp. olive oil
- Four large tomatoes, chopped
- Two tsp. herbs de Provence

Directions:

Blend the basil, parsley, coriander, mint, lemon juice and capers, with a little salt and pepper. Make sure all Ingredients are well incorporated

Preheat and set the temperature at 400 F (204 C)

Coat the eggplant, onion, garlic, pepper, fennel, and zucchini with olive oil.

Transfer the vegetable into the baking dish and top with the tomatoes and herb puree. Sprinkle with more salt and pepper, and the herbs de Provence

Place the baking dish into rack position 1, select convection bake and set time to 26 minutes

Serve immediately

Nutrition:

Energy (calories): 358 kcal

Protein: 6.99 g

Fat: 19.36 g

Carbohydrates: 45.8 g

Potato and Broccoli with Tofu Scramble

Preparation time: 15 minutes
Cooking time: 30 minutes
Servings: 3

Ingredients:

- 2 ½ cups chopped red potato
- Two tbsp. olive oil, divided
- One block tofu, chopped finely
- Two tbsp. tamari
- One tsp. turmeric powder
- ½ tsp. garlic powder
- ½ cup chopped onion
- 4 cups broccoli florets

Directions:

Preheat and set the temperature at 400 F (204 C)

Toss together the potatoes and one tbsp. of the olive oil, then transfer to a baking dish

Place the baking dish into Rack position 1, select convention Bake and set time to 15 minutes. Stir the potatoes once during cooking

Combine the tofu, the remaining one tbsp. of the olive oil, turmeric, onion powder, tamari, and garlic powder, stirring in the onions, followed by the broccoli

Top the potatoes with the tofu mixture and bake for an additional 15 minutes

Serve warm

Nutrition:

Energy (calories): 220 kcal

Protein: 11.88 g

Fat: 11.41 g

Carbohydrates: 20.77 g

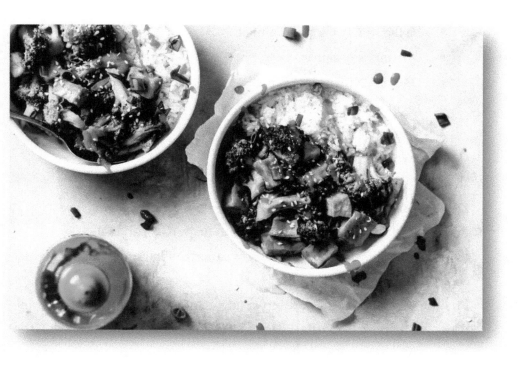

Lush Summer Rolls

Preparation time: 15 minutes
Cooking time: 15 minutes
Servings: 4

Ingredients:

- 1 cup shiitake mushroom, sliced thinly
- One celery stalk, chopped
- One medium carrot, shredded
- ½ tsp. finely chopped ginger
- One tsp. soy sauce
- One tsp. Nutritional yeast
- Eight spring roll sheets
- One tsp. corn water
- Two tbsp. water

Directions:

Preheat and set the temperature at 400 degrees F (204 C)

In a bowl, combine the ginger, soy sauce, Nutritional yeast, carrots, celery, mushroom, and sugar

Mix the cornstarch and water to create an adhesive for the spring rolls

Scoop a tbsp. full of the vegetable mixture into the middle of the spring roll sheets. Brush the edges of the sheets with the cornstarch adhesive and enclose around the filling to make spring rolls. Arrange the rolls in the air fryer basket

Place the air fryer basket on the baking pan and move into position 2 of the rack; choose Air Fry and set the time to 15 minutes or until crisp.

Serve hot

Nutrition:

Energy (calories): 250 kcal

Protein: 8.99 g

Fat: 3.47 g

Carbohydrates: 45.04 g

Super Veg Rolls

Preparation time: 20 minutes

Cooking time: 10 minutes

Servings: 6

Ingredients:

- Two potatoes, mashed
- ¼ cup peas
- ½ cup mashed carrots
- One small cabbage, sliced
- ¼ cups beans
- Two tbsp. sweet corn
- One small onion, chopped
- ½ cup bread crumbs
- One packet spring roll sheets
- ½ cup cornstarch slurry

Directions:

Preheat and set the temperature at 390 F (199 C)

Boil all the vegetables in water over low heat. Rinse and allow drying

Unroll the spring roll sheets and spoon equal amounts of vegetables onto the center of each one. Fold into spring tools and coat each one with the slurry and bread crumbs. Transfer to the air fryer basket

Place on the baking pan the air fryer basket and slide into rack position2; pick Air Fry and set the time to 10 minutes

Serve warm

Nutrition:

Energy (calories): 202 kcal

Protein: 5.1 g

Fat: 0.69 g

Carbohydrates: 45.4 g

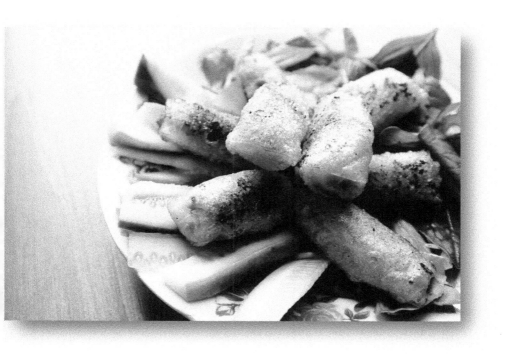

Sweet Potatoes with Tofu

Preparation time: 15 minutes

Cooking time: 35 minutes

Servings: 8

Ingredients:

- Eight sweet potatoes, scrubbed
- Two tbsp. olive oil
- One large onion, chopped
- Two green chillies, deseeded and chopped
- 8 ounces (227 g) tofu, crumbled
- Two tbsp. Cajun seasoning
- 1 cup chopped tomatoe s
- One can of kidney beans, must drained and rinsed
- Salt and ground black pepper, to taste

Directions:

Preheat and set the temperature at 400 F (204 C)

With a knife, pierce the skin of the sweet potatoes and transfer them to the air fryer basket

Place the air fryer basket onto the baking pan and slide into Rack position 2. Select air fry and set time to 30 minutes, or until soft.

Remove from the oven, halve each potato, and set to one side

Over medium heat, fry the onions and chillies in the olive oil in a skillet for 2 minutes until fragrant

Add the tofu and Cajun seasoning and air fry for a further 3 minutes before incorporating the kidney beans and tomatoes. Sprinkle some salt and pepper as desire

Top each sweet potato halves with a spoonful of the tofu mixture and serve

Nutrition:

Energy (calories): 127 kcal

Protein: 5.45 g

Fat: 9.16 g

Carbohydrates: 7.22 g

Rice and Eggplant Bowl

Preparation time: 15 minutes

Cooking time: 10 minutes

Servings: 4

Ingredients:

- ¼ cup sliced cucumber
- One tsp. salt
- One tbsp. sugar
- Seven tbsp. Japanese rice vinegar
- Three medium eggplants, sliced
- Three tbsp. sweet white miso paste
- One tbsp. mirin rice wine
- 4 cups cooked sushi rice
- Four spring onions
- One tbsp. toasted sesame seeds

Directions:

Coat the cucumber slices with the rice wine vinegar, salt, and sugar

Put a dish on top of the bowl to weight it down completely

In a bowl, mix the eggplants, mirin rice wine, and miso paste. Allow marinating for half an hour

Preheat and set the temperature at 400 F (204 C)

Slice the eggplant and put in the air fryer basket

Place the air fryer basket onto the baking pan and slide into rack position 2, select air fry and set time to 10 minutes

Fill the bottom of a serving bowl with rice and top with the eggplants and pickled cucumbers

Add the spring onions and sesame seeds for garnish. Serve immediately

Nutrition:

Energy (calories): 516 kcal

Protein: 20.82 g

Fat: 26.82 g

Carbohydrates: 88.75 g

Cauliflower, Chickpea, and Avocado Mash

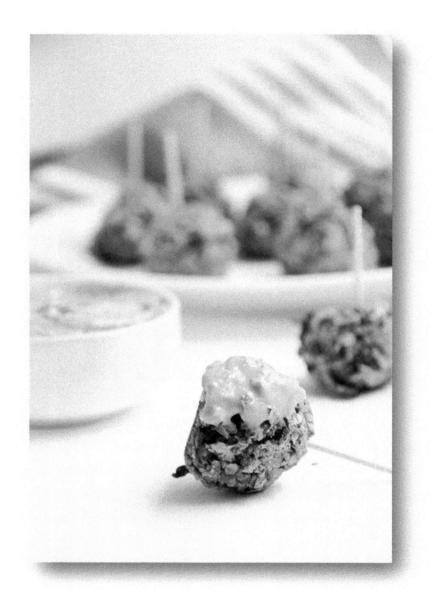

Preparation time: 10 minutes

Cooking time: 25 minutes

Servings: 4

Ingredients:

- One medium head cauliflower, cut into florets
- One can chickpeas, drained and rinsed
- One tbsp. extra-virgin olive oil
- Two tbsp. lemon juice
- Salt and ground pepper, to taste
- Four flatbreads, toasted
- Two ripe avocados, mashed

Directions:

Preheat and set the temperature at 425 F (218 C)

In a bowl, mix the chickpeas, cauliflower, lemon juice and olive oil. Sprinkle salt and pepper as desired. Transfer to the air fryer basket

Place the air fryer basket onto the baking pan and slide into Rack position 2, select air fry and set time to 25 minutes

Spread on top of the flatbread with the mashed avocado. Sprinkle with more pepper and salt and serve

Nutrition:

Energy (calories): 285 kcal

Protein: 7.96 g

Fat: 18.04 g

Carbohydrates: 28.03 g

Mushroom and Pepper Pizza Squares

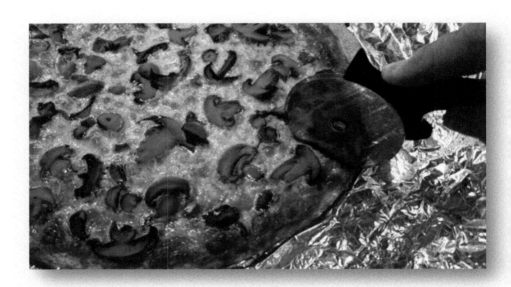

Preparation time: 10 minutes

Cooking time: 10 minutes

Servings: 10

Ingredients:

- One pizza dough, cut into squares
- 1 cup chopped oyster mushrooms
- One shallot, chopped
- ¼ red bell pepper, chopped
- Two tbsp. parsley

- Salt and ground black pepper to taste

Directions:

Preheat and set the temperature at 400 F (204 c)

In a bowl, combine the oyster mushrooms, shallot, bell pepper and parsley. Sprinkle some salt and pepper as desired

Spread the mixture on top of the pizza squares, and then transfer to a baking pan

Slide the baking pan into Rack position 1, select convection bake and set time to 10 minutes

Serve warm.

Nutrition:

Energy (calories): 161 kcal

Protein: 7.8 g

Fat: 5.28 g

Carbohydrates: 20.85 g

Balsamic Brussels Sprouts

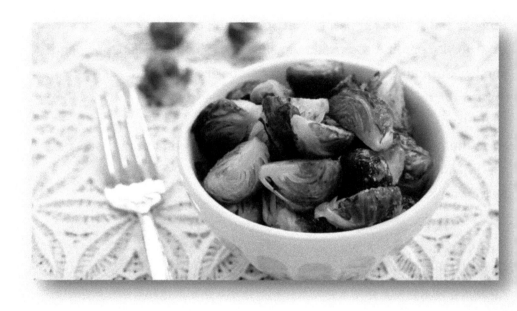

Preparation time: 5 minutes

Cooking time: 13 minutes

Servings: 2

Ingredients:

- 2 cups Brussels sprouts, halved
- One tbsp. olive oil
- One tbsp. balsamic vinegar
- One tbsp. maple syrup
- ¼ tsp. of sea salt

Directions:

Preheat and set the temperature at 375 F (191 C)

Evenly coat the brussels sprouts with olive oil, balsamic vinegar, maple syrup, and salt. Transfer to the air fryer basket

Place the air fryer basket onto the baking pan and slide into Rack position 2, select air fry and set time to 5 minutes

Give the basket a good shake, increase the temperature to 400 F (204 C) and continue to air fry for another 8 minutes

Serve hot.

Nutrition:

Energy (calories): 131 kcal

Protein: 3.02 g

Fat: 7.02 g

Carbohydrates: 15.94 g

Green Beans with Shallot

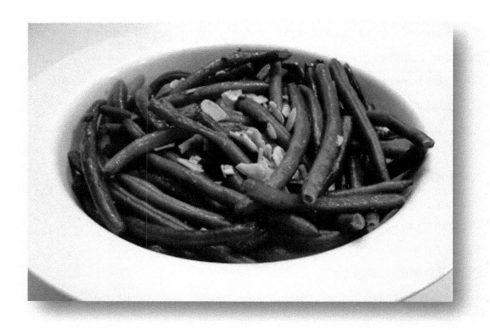

Preparation time: 10 minutes

Cooking time: 10 minutes

Servings: 4

Ingredients:

- 1 ½ pound (680 g) French green beans, stems removed and blanched
- One tbsp. salt
- ½ pound (227 g) shallots, peeled and cut into quatres
- ½ tsp. ground white pepper

25

- Two tbsp. olive oil

Directions:

Preheat and set the temperature at 400 F (204 C)

Coat the vegetables with the rest of the Ingredients in a bowl. Transfer to the air fryer basket

Place the air fryer basket onto baking pan and slide rack position 2, select air fry and set time 10 minutes, making sure the green beans achieve a light brown colour

Serve hot

Nutrition:

Energy (calories): 166 kcal

Protein: 3.91 g

Fat: 7.16 g

Carbohydrates: 22.49 g

Black Bean and Tomato Chili

Preparation time: 15 minutes

Cooking time: 23 minutes

Servings: 6

Ingredients:

- One tbsp. olive oil
- One medium onion, diced
- Three garlic cloves, minced
- 1 cup vegetable brot h
- Three cans of black beans must drained and rinsed
- Two cans of diced tomatoes
- Two chipotle peppers, chopped
- Two tsp. chilli powder
- One tsp. dried oregano
- ½ tsp. salt

Directions:

Over medium heat, fry the garlic add onion in the olive oil for 3 minutes

Add the remaining Ingredients, stirring constantly and scraping the bottom to prevent sticking

Preheat and set the temperature at 400 F (204 C)

Take a dish and place the mixture inside. On top put a sheet of aluminum foil.

Place the dish into Rack Position 1, select convection bake and set time to 20 minutes

Serve immediately

Nutrition:

Energy (calories): 362 kcal

Protein: 1.27 g

Fat: 38.95 g

Carbohydrates: 6.52 g

Herbed Pita Chips

Preparation time: 5 minutes
Cooking time: 6 minutes
Servings: 4

Ingredients:

- ¼ tsp. dried basil
- ¼ tsp. marjoram
- ¼ tsp. ground oregano
- ¼ tsp. garlic powder
- ¼ tsp. ground thyme
- ¼ tsp. salt
- ¼ tsp. salt
- Two whole 6-inch pitas, whole grain or white cooking spray

Directions:

Preheat and set the temperature at 330 F

Mix all the seasoning

Cut each pita half into four wedges; break apart wedges at the fold

Mist one side of pita wedges with oil. Sprinkle with half of the seasoning mix.

Turn pita wedges over, mist the other side with oil, and sprinkle with remaining seasoning. Place the pita wedges in a baking pan

Slide the baking pan into rack position 1, select convention bake and set time to 4 minutes. Shake the pan in the middle of **Cooking time**

If needed, bake for 1 or 2 more minutes until crisp. Serve hot

Nutrition:

Energy (calories): 485 kcal

Protein: 17.9 g

Fat: 4.74 g

Carbohydrates: 100.36 g

Lemony Pear Chips

Preparation time: 15 minutes

Cooking time: 12 minutes

Servings: 4

Ingredients:

- Two firm bosc pears, cut crosswise into 1/8-inch-thick slices
- One tbsp. freshly squeezed lemon juice
- ½ tsp. ground cinnamon
- 1/8 tsp. ground cardamom

Directions:

Preheat and set the temperature at 380 F

Separate the smaller stem-end pear rounds from the large rounds with seeds. Remove the core and seeds from the large slices. Sprinkle all slices with lemon juice, cinnamon, and cardamom

Put the smaller chips into the air fryer basket

Place the air fryer basket onto the baking pan and slide into rack position 2; select air fryer and set time to 5 minutes, or until light golden brown. Shake the basket once during cooking. Remove from the oven.

Repeat with the larger slices, air frying for 6 to 8 minutes, or until light golden brown, shaking the basket once during cooking

Remove the chips from the oven, cool and serve or store in an airtight container at room temperature up for two days

Nutrition:

Energy (calories): 62 kcal

Protein: 0.36 g

Fat: 0.1 g

Carbohydrates: 14.99 g

Artichoke Pesto Pasta With Air-Fried Chickpeas

Preparation time: 10 minutes

Cooking time: 15 minutes

Servings: 4

Ingredients:

- 8 ounces vegan pappardelle or other pasta
- One packed cup (1 ounce) fresh basil leaves
- Six jarred artichoke hearts drained and squeezed slightly to remove excess liquid
- 2 Tbsp. shelled pumpkin seeds (pepitas)
- Juice of half a lemon (~1 Tbsp.)
- One clove garlic
- ½ tsp. white miso paste
- One tsp. extra virgin olive oil (optional)
- One batch air-fried or roasted chickpeas

Directions:

Cook the pasta according to package Directions.

While pasta is cooking, you can combine basil leaves, artichoke hearts, shelled pumpkin seeds, lemon juice, garlic, and white miso paste in a food processor until it is thoroughly combined. Scrape down the sides, as needed, and then continue processing until the pesto is mostly smooth.

If the pasta is already cooked, drain in a colander. Then transfer the noodles to a larger bowl and add extra virgin olive oil to keep them from sticking together (optional). Spoon over the pasta with the artichoke pesto, and toss until evenly mixed.

Serve pasta topped with chickpeas which are air-fried or roasted.

Nutrition:

Energy (calories): 196 kcal

Protein: 7.96 g

Fat: 3.38 g

Carbohydrates: 38.74 g

Fishless Tacos With Chipotle Crema

Preparation time: 10 minutes

Cooking time: 20 minutes

Servings: 4

Ingredients:

- For the tacos:
- 6 Gardein fishless filets
- Six soft corn tortillas
- 1 ½ cups chopped green leaf lettuce or Romaine
- 3 Tbsp. chopped onions
- Two avocados, pit removed and sliced
- Cilantro, chopped (garnish)
- One lime, sliced (for serving)
- For the chipotle crema:
- ½ cup + 1 Tbsp. raw cashews
- ¾ cup of water (plus extra for soaking, if not using a high-speed blender)
- Two chipotle peppers in adobo sauce (from 7 oz. can)
- One tsp. adobo sauce from a can
- One tsp. agave syrup
- ½ tsp. lemon juice
- 1/8 tsp. salt

Directions:

To make the tacos:

Cook the Gardein fishless filets see Directions on the package.

In a prepared skillet, warm the corn tortillas one at a time for about 1 minute on each side on medium heat. If each tortilla has been warmed on both sides, move it to a plate and then cover with a clean dish towel to keep them pliable until serving.

Once the filets are fully cooked, remove them from the oven and slice them into four pieces on a bias. Put a sliced filet in each tortilla and stuff with green leaf lettuce, onions, sliced avocado, and a sprinkling of cilantro. Drizzle each taco with chipotle crema and then serve with lime slices.

To make the chipotle crema:

If you don›t have a high-speed blender, soak the cashews in water for several hours, and then drain. If you will use a high-speed blender, you can skip this step.

Put the cashews, ¾ cup water, chipotle peppers, adobo sauce, agave syrup, and lemon juice in a blender. Blend until smooth. For 24 hours, it'll be the best. (If you are helping the crema right away and don't have time, try reducing the amount of water by a tbsp...)

Nutrition:

Energy (calories): 465 kcal

Protein: 8.64 g

Fat: 33.76 g

Carbohydrates: 39.9 g

Easy Vegan Falafel

Preparation time: 10 minutes

Cooking time: 15 minutes

Servings: 4

Ingredients:

- One 15-ounce (425 g) can chickpeas, rinsed, drained and patted dry
- 1/3 Cup (15 g) of chopped fresh parsley (or sub cilantro)
- Four cloves garlic, minced
- Two shallots, minced (3/4cup, 65 g | or sub white onion)
- 2 Tbsp. (17 g) of raw sesame seeds or you can use (sub finely chopped nuts, such as pecans)
- 1 ½ tsp. cumin, plus more to taste
- ¼ tsp. sea salt
- black pepper
- Optional: A Healthy pinch each cardamom and coriander
- 3-4 Tbsp. (24-31 g) all-purpose flour (or use as sub oat flour or gluten-free blend with varied results)
- 3-4 tbsp. (45 - 60 ml) of grapeseed oil for cooking (or use any neutral oil with a high smoke point)
- Optional: Panko bread crumbs for coating (see pacakge for instructions)
- Garlic Dill Sauce for serving

Directions:

In a food processor or blender, add the chickpeas, parsley, sesame seeds, shallot, garlic, cumin, salt, pepper (and coriander and cardamom if used) and mix/pulse to combine, scraping down the sides as needed until thoroughly combined.

Add one tbsp. of flour at a time and pulse/mix until the dough is no longer wet, and you can shape the dough into a ball without sticking to your hands - I used 4 Tbsp. Taste the seasonings and change them as needed. I added a little more salt, pepper, and a splash of coriander and cardamom.

To firm up, move to a mixing bowl, cover and refrigerate for 1-2 hours. You can skip this step if you're in a rush, but they'll be a little more delicate when cooking.

Once chilled, scoop out rounded tbsp. amounts (30 g in weight / I used scoop) and gently form into 11-12 small discs.

Optional: Sprinkle with panko bread crumbs and press to stick gently - turn and repeat. This is going to create a crispier crust, but this is optional.

Heat a large skillet over medium heat and add enough oil to coat the pan - about 2 Tbsp. generously. Swirl to coat.

If the oil is hot, add only as many falafels as will fit very comfortably in the pan at a time - about

Cook for 4-5 minutes in all, flipping when deep golden brown is on the underside. The deeper golden brown they are, the crispier they will be, repeat until all falafel is browned. When slightly cooled, they will also firm up further.

Serve warm with garlic-dill sauce or hummus, inside a pita with desired toppings or atop a greens bed.

Best when fresh, while leftovers can be kept covered for several days in the refrigerator. Freeze after that for up to 1 month to remain new.

Nutrition:

Energy (calories): 347 kcal

Protein: 10.54 g

Fat: 18 g

Carbohydrates: 37.48 g

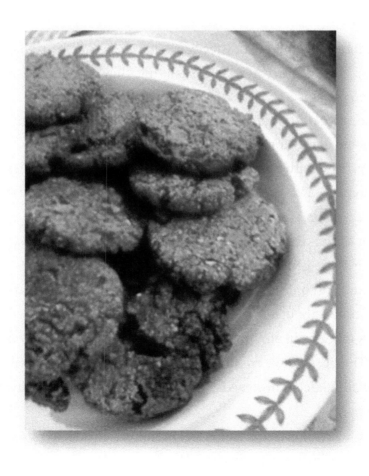

Thai-Style Vegan Crab Cakes

Preparation time: 10 minutes
Cooking time: 15 minutes
Servings: 4

Ingredients:

- 600g / 4 cups diced or about four medium potatoes
- 7-8 individual / 1 bunch green onions
- One lime, zest & juice
- 1½ inch knob of fresh ginger
- One tbsp. Tamari, or soy sauce
- Four tbsp. Thai Red Curry Paste
- Four sheets nori
- 220g / 1 can heart of palm; the long tubular shaped ones work best
- 100g / ¾ cup canned artichoke hearts
- pepper, to tast e
- salt, to taste
- Two tbsp. oil for pan-frying, optional
-

Directions:

The potatoes are peeled and cubed, then added to a pan. Cover and fork-tender with water and simmer, then rinse, mash and set aside.

When the potatoes are boiling, add a food processor with the green onions, lime juice, lime zest, ginger, tamari and curry paste. Break the nori sheets into manageable pieces and place them with the other Ingredients in the food processor. Process until a paste is made. The nori appears to remain a little bit more chunky than everything else, and that's all right.

Drain the hearts of palm, either grate them or shred them with a fork, then drain the artichokes and roughly chop.

When the potatoes are sufficiently cooled to handle, add the pasta and mix well so it is evenly distributed, then add the shredded palm hearts and the chopped artichoke and gently stir through.

Shape them into patties and put them as you go on a tray with some baking parchment. You can either pan-fry them for cooking, bake them in the oven or cook them on a griddle. As they grow a lovely golden crust, they are best pan-fried.

To pan-fry

Warm a couple tbsp. of oil in a pan at set medium-high heat. Once really hot, add the crab cakes carefully. To allow a dense, golden crust to develop, leave them well alone for about 4 minutes, then turn over and do the same on the other side. To absorb excess oil, remove it from the pan and rest it on some kitchen paper. Your pan can not be large enough to cook all of them at once, so have the oven low and pop the cooked ones in there to keep the others warm while you cook.

To griddle

Warm your griddle to medium-high heat. When hot, carefully place the crab cakes on the griddle and cook for 4-5 minutes on each side.

To oven bake

Place on a tray on baking parchment and bake at 400°F for around 25 minutes. Turn over halfway through.

Nutrition:

Energy (calories): 477 kcal

Protein: 11.6 g

Fat: 8.96 g

Carbohydrates: 94.02 g

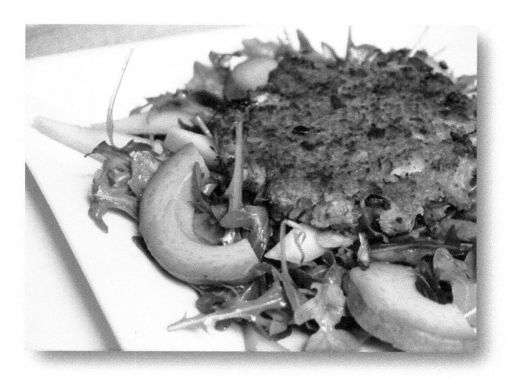

Almond-Crusted Cauliflower Bites with Avocado Ranch Dip

Preparation time: 10 minutes

Cooking time: 15 minutes

Servings: 4

Ingredients:

- Avocado Ranch Dip
- 1 cup heaping mashed avocado
- Two tbsp. unsweetened non-dairy milk
- One tbsp. white vinegar
- One tbsp. lemon juice
- ½ tsp. onion powder
- ½ tsp. dried parsley
- ½ tsp. Nutritional yeast
- ¼-½ tsp. sea salt to taste
- ¼ tsp. garlic powder
- ¼ tsp. agave nectar
- Pinch of dried dill
- Almond-crusted Cauliflower Bites
- One piece large head cauliflower florets chopped into bite-sized
- ½ cup unsweetened non-dairy milk
- Six tbsp. vegan mayo soy-free

- ¼ cup chickpea flour
- ¾ cup almond meal
- ¼ cup cornmeal
- One tsp. onion powder
- One tsp. garlic powder
- One tsp. of sea salt
- ½ tsp. paprika
- Pinch of black pepper

Directions:

Place all Ingredients in a prepared mixing bowl and mash together until combined and mostly smooth. Refrigerate until ready to serve.

Almond-crusted Cauliflower Bites

Preheat oven at temeprature of 400F and line a large baking sheet with parchment paper or a silicone mat .

Whisk together the non-dairy milk, vegan mayo and chickpea flour in a medium mixing bowl until smooth and thick enough to cover a spoon. Mix the almond meal, cornmeal, onion powder, garlic powder, salt, paprika and pepper in another mixing bowl until mixed.

Take each piece of cauliflower and first dunk it into the wet mixture, let excess drip off, then press into crumb mixture, covering evenly and shaking off loose bits; place onto the a baking sheet. Repeat until all pieces are coated and then on the baking sheet.

Coat cauliflower bites lightly with cooking oil spray and place in oven. Bake for 15 minutes, flip pieces over and lightly spray with oil again, bake for an additional 15 minutes or until golden. The cool baking sheet on a rack for 5 minutes before serving with avocado ranch dip!

Nutrition:

Energy (calories): 485 kcal

Protein: 7.67 g

Fat: 41.41 g

Carbohydrates: 25.66 g

Simple Vegan Spring Rolls

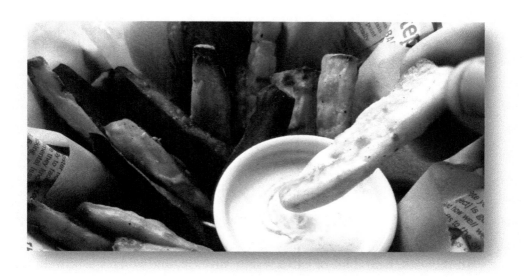

Preparation time: 10 minutes

Cooking time: 15 minutes

Servings: 4

Ingredients:

- Extra virgin olive oil
- Four cloves of garlic
- One onion
- Two carrots
- Four leaves of cabbage
- 1 ounce or 30 grams soy sprouts

Two tbsp. tamari or soy sauce

Eight sheets spring roll pastry

Water

Sweet and sour sauce

Directions:

In a wok, heat extra virgin olive oil (1 tbsp. is sufficient), add the vegetables (garlic, julienne, carrots, cabbage, and soy sprouts) and the tamari sauce. Cook over a medium-high heat for around 5 minutes...

You can see how to make the vegan spring rolls in the sixth photo of this post. You only have to place the wrapper like a diamond, place two tbsp. of filling near a corner, tightly roll the wrapper, fold over the left side, fold over the right side, paint a little water along the edge and close it up.

In the wok, heat a lot of extra virgin olive oil, and when it's scorching, add the spring rolls and cook for around 1 minute or until golden brown on both sides.

Nutrition:

Energy (calories): 285 kcal

Protein: 9.66 g

Fat: 4.72 g

Carbohydrates: 50.6 g

Vegan Popcorn

Preparation time: 10 minutes

Cooking time: 15 minutes

Servings: 4

Ingredients:

- 2 cups dried soy chunks
- 3 cups vegetable broth
- Two cloves of garlic, mashed
- 1 tsp. salt
- 1-inch cube of ginger, grated
- ½ cup flour
- ¾ cup vegetable broth
- ½ cup cornstarch
- 1 cup bread crumbs
- 1 tbsp. garlic powder
- 1 tbsp. lemon pepper
- ½ tsp. salt
- For the dip:
- 1 tbsp. chopped fresh dill
- 1/3 Cup sour cream (use sour soy cream to keep it vegan)
- dash of salt and pepper

Directions:

Combine soy chunks, ginger, mashed garlic, 1 tsp. of salt, and fill the bowl with vegetable broth in a wide bowl until the soy chunks are coated. Soak until the bits are soft, or about 20 minutes.

Heat a pot with an inch of oil on medium-high heat.

Mix ½ cup flour and ¾ cup vegetable broth from the soaking soy chunks and whisk until no lumps remain—divide between two bowls .

Squeeze the excess fluid from the soy chunks gently and coat in one of the bowls of the flour mixture until the chunks are soft and soaked.

Using 1/2 cup cornstarch to move the chunks to a Ziploc bag. Shake until coated, then move to the second bowl of flour mixture, cover, and then place the garlic powder, bread crumbs, lemon pepper, and salt in another ziploc container.

In batches, fry the chunks in oil until golden. To fry both sides, you can need to shift them around because they seem to like to float in one direction.

Remove and drain on a sheet of paper towel.

In a food processor, blend the dill, sour cream, salt and pepper to make the dip.

Serve the fried chunks with dip and enjoy!

Nutrition:

Energy (calories): 1676 kcal

Protein: 15.79 g

Fat: 166.67 g

Carbohydrates: 45.24 g

Stuffed Baby Eggplant

Air Fryer Stuffed Baby Eggplant is a delicious Indian dish made with baby eggplants packed full of aromatic and flavorful spices. This dish makes the perfect appetizer or first course for an elegant dinner.

Preparation time: 8 minutes
Cooking time: 12 minutes
Servings: 4

Ingredients:
- For the eggplant:
- Eight baby eggplants rinsed and patted dry
- 2 tsp. olive oil
- For the spice stuffing:
- 1 tsp. Ground cumin
- ¾ tbsp. Coriander powder
- ¾ tbsp. Dry mango powder
- ½ tsp. Ground turmeric
- ½ tsp. Kashmiri red chilli powder
- ½ tsp. garlic powder
- 1 tsp. salt
- To Garnish:
- 1 tbsp. cilantro leaves to garnish

Directions:

In a small bowl, stir all the stuffing spice together.

Take the eggplants and leaving the stems intact. Slit in the center from the bottom until just above the branch, careful not to split the eggplant into two pieces.

Now turn the eggplant at 90 degrees and add another slit from the center. The eggplant should in 4 but still held together by the stem.

Mix a tsp. of oil in the spices, and with a small spoon, fills the spice paste into each slit of the eggplants.

In the air fryer, put the eggplants in a single layer and brush oil on each eggplant, ensuring that both sides are coated...

Cook the air fryer at 360 degrees Fahrenheit for 8-12 minutes.

The colour will change when they are cooked. At 8 minutes, check the eggplant, and cook for additional time as needed.

Garnish with cilantro, and enjoy!

Nutrition:

Calories: 106 kcal.

Total Carbohydrates 20g

Protein 3g

Total Fat 3g

Potassium 679mg

Vegan Fruits

Easy Pears Dessert

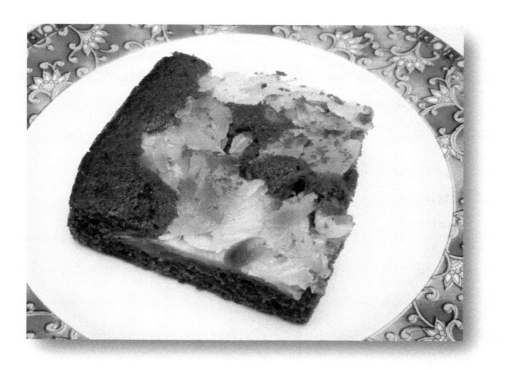

Preparation time: 10 minutes

Cooking time: 25 minutes

Servings: 12

Ingredients:

- Six big pears, cored and chopped
- ½ cup raisins
- One tsp. ginger powder
- ¼ cup of coconut sugar
- One tsp. lemon zest, grated

Directions:

In a pan that exactly on your air fryer, mix pears with raisins, ginger, sugar and lemon zest, stir, introduce in the fryer and cook at 350 degrees F for 25 minutes.

Divide into bowls and serve cold.

Enjoy!

Nutrition:

Calories 200

Fat 3g

Fibre 4g

Carbs 6g

Protein 6g

Vanilla Strawberry Mix

Preparation time: 10 minutes

Cooking time: 20 minutes

Servings: 10

Ingredients:

- Two tbsp. lemon juice
- 2 pounds of strawberries
- 4 cups of coconut sugar
- One tsp. cinnamon powder
- One tsp. vanilla extract

Directions:

In a pan that exactly on your air fryer, mix strawberries with coconut sugar, lemon juice, cinnamon and vanilla, stir gently, introduce in the fryer and cook at 350 degrees F for 20 minutes

Divide into bowls and serve cold.

Enjoy!

Nutrition:

Calories 140

Fat 0g

Fibre 1g

Carbs 5g

Protein 2g

Sweet Bananas and Sauce

Preparation time: 10 minutes

Cooking time: 20 minutes

Servings: 2

Ingredients:

- Juice of ½ lemon
- 3 tbsp. agave nectar
- 1 tbsp. coconut oil
- 4 bananas, peeled and sliced diagonally
- ½ tsp. cardamom seeds

Directions:

Arrange bananas in a pan that fits your air fryer, add agave nectar, lemon juice, oil and cardamom, introduce in the fryer and cook at 360 degrees F for 20 minutes

Divide bananas and sauce between plates and serve.

Enjoy!

Nutrition:

calories 210

Fat 1g

Fiber 2g

Carbs 8g

Protein 3g

Vegan Dessert

Cozy Apple Crisp

Preparation time: 10 minutes

Cooking time: 30 minutes

Servings: 4

Bake: 320°F

Ingredients:

- For the topping
- 2 tbsps. coconut oil
- ¼ cup plus 2 tbsps. whole-wheat pastry flour (or gluten-free all-purpose flour)
- ¼ cup of coconut sugar
- 1/8 Tsp. sea salt
- For the filling
- 2 cups finely chopped (or thinly sliced) apples (no need to peel)
- 3 tbsp. water
- ½ tbsp. lemon juice
- ¾ tsp. cinnamon

Directions:

To make the topping:

In a bowl, combine the oil, flour, sugar, and salt. Mix the Ingredients thoroughly, either with your hands or a spoon. The mixture should be crumbly; if it's not, place it in the fridge until it solidifies a bit.

To make the filling:

In a 6-inch round, 2-inch deep baking pan, stir the apples with the water, lemon juice, and cinnamon until well combined.

Crumble the chilled topping over the apples. Bake for 30 minutes, or until the apples are tender and the crumble is crunchy and nicely browned. Serve immediately on its own or topped with nondairy milk, vegan ice cream, or non-dairy whipped cream.

Variation Tip: My daughter and I both love this dessert but disagree on what constitutes the best crumble topping. I prefer the one that's written in the recipe above. However, she prefers a more decadent version that includes vegan margarine and regular sugar. If you'd like to try her performance (and she strongly suggests you do), replace the coconut oil with vegan margarine and the coconut sugar with organic white sugar.

Ingredient Tip: I'm often asked what type of apples work best in this recipe. And in all honesty, I don't have an impressive answer—I tend to search out the best-looking organic apples at the store. As long as they're not overly tart, most varieties will work wonderfully.

Nutrition:

Calories: 172
Total fat: 7g
Cholesterol: 0mg

Carbohydrates: 29g

Fibre: 4g

Protein: 1g

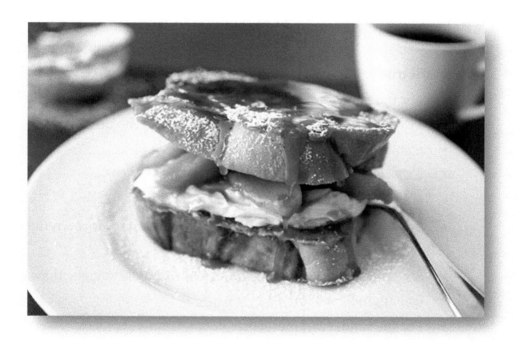

Apple Puffs with Vanilla Caramel Sauce

Preparation time: 20 minutes

Cooking time: 10 minutes

Servings: 6 puffs

Bake: 320°F

Ingredients:

- For the filling:
- Two medium apples, cored and finely diced (no need to peel)
- 2 tsp. cinnamon
- 2 tbsps. coconut sugar
- 1/8 tsp. sea salt
- Cooking oil spray it can be (sunflower, safflower, or refined coconut)
- Six large (13-inch x 17-inch) sheets of phyllo dough, thawed (see Ingredient Tip)
- For the vanilla caramel sauce:
- A 6-inch segment of a vanilla bean
- ½ cup plus one tbsp. maple syrup
- ¼ cup plus two tbsp. refined coconut oil (or vegan margarine)
- ¼ cup of coconut sugar
- ½ tsp. of sea salt

Directions:

To make the filling:

In a prepared medium bowl, combine the apples, cinnamon, coconut sugar, and salt and set aside.

Spray the air fryer basket with oil spray and set aside. Gently unwrap the phyllo dough. Remove six sheets and carefully set them aside. Wrap the remaining phyllo in airtight plastic wrap and place back in the fridge.

To assemble the puffs:

Remove one large sheet of phyllo and place it on a clean, dry surface. Spray with the oil. Fold it into thirds (the long way, so that you form a long, skinny rectangle). As you go, spray each portion of dry phyllo so the exposed phyllo continually gets lightly coated with oil—this will give you a more flaky (vs. dry) result.

Place 1/3 cup of the apple mixture at the base of the phyllo rectangle. Fold the bottom of the phyllo up and over the mixture. Continue to fold up toward the top, forming it into a triangle as you go. Once you have an apple-filled triangle, place it in the air fryer basket and spray the top with oil.

Repeat with the remaining phyllo and apple mixture. Note: You'll probably only be able to fit three puffs in your air fryer at a time because you don't want them to overlap. If you don't wish to make a second batch right now, store the phyllo-wrapped, uncooked puffs in an airtight container and put in the fridge and air-fry them within a day or two.

Bake for 10 minutes, or until very golden-browned.

To make the sauce:

Make a lengthwise cut down the vanilla bean with a sharp knife and pry it open. Scrape out the insides with a table knife and place in a small pot. Add the maple syrup, oil, coconut sugar, and salt to the pot and set to medium-low heat, stirring very well to combine. After the sauce comes to a boil, reduce the heat to low and simmer gently for 3 to 5 minutes or slightly thickened.

Transfer the apple puffs to a plate and top with the caramel sauce. Enjoy while warm.

Ingredient Tip: Phyllo (aka filo) dough is easy to use, so don't be intimidated! There are just a few things you need to know: First, be sure to thaw frozen packages in the fridge overnight. I don't find it necessary to cover the unwrapped dough with damp towels, as most recipes suggest—just have the filling ready to go, and then work quickly once you've opened the package. And of course, be very gentle when working with phyllo, as it tears easily—but if it does pull, just place another sheet on top (or "patch" it with additional phyllo), and no one will ever know!

Nutrition:

Calories: 366

Total fat: 16g

Cholesterol: 0mg

Carbohydrates: 58g

Fibre: 3g

Protein: 2g

Strawberry Puffs with Creamy Lemon Sauce

Preparation time: 20 minutes

Cooking time: 10 minutes

Servings: 8 puffs

Bake: 320°F

Ingredients:

- For the filling
- 3 cups sliced strawberries, fresh or frozen (1½ pints or 24 ounces)
- 1 cup sugar-free strawberry jam (sweetened only with fruit juice)
- 1 tbsp. arrowroot (or cornstarch)
- Cooking oil spray it can be (sunflower, safflower, or refined coconut)
- Eight large (13-inch x 17-inch) sheets of phyllo dough, thawed (see Ingredient Tip)
- For the sauce
- 1 cup raw cashew pieces (see Cooking Tip)
- ¼ cup plus 2 tbsp. raw agave nectar
- ¼ cup plus 1 tbsp. water
- 3 tbsp. fresh lemon juice
- 2 tsp. (packed) lemon zest (see Cooking Tip)

- 2 tbsp. neutral-flavoured oil (sunflower, safflower, or refined coconut)
- 2 tsp. vanilla
- ¼ tsp. of sea salt

Directions:

To make the filling:

In a medium bowl, add the strawberries, jam, and arrowroot and stir well to combine. Set aside.

Spray the air fryer basket using oil spray and set aside.

To assemble the puffs:

Gently unwrap the phyllo dough. Remove eight sheets and carefully set them aside. Re-wrap the remaining phyllo in airtight plastic wrap and place it back in the fridge.

Remove one large sheet of phyllo and place it on a clean, dry surface. Spray with the oil. Fold it into thirds so that it forms a long, skinny rectangle. As you go, spray each portion of dry phyllo so the exposed phyllo continually gets lightly coated with oil.

Place about 1/3 cup of the strawberry mixture at the base of the phyllo rectangle. Fold the bottom of the phyllo up and over the mixture. Continue to fold up toward the top, forming it into a triangle as you go. Once fully wrapped, place it in the air fryer basket and spray the top with oil.

Repeat with the remaining phyllo and strawberry mixture. Note you'll probably only be able to fit three puffs in your air fryer at a time because you don't want them to overlap.

Bake for 10 minutes, or until beautifully golden-browned.

To make the sauce:

Place the cashews, agave, water, lemon juice and zest, oil, vanilla, and salt in a blender. Process until completely smooth and velvety. (Any leftover sauce will keep nicely in the fridge for up to a week.)

Transfer the strawberry puffs to a plate and drizzle with the creamy lemon sauce. If desired, garnish with sliced strawberries. Enjoy while warm.

Cooking Tip: If your blender isn't a high-speed one (such as Vitamix or Blendtec), you'll need to soak the cashews in sufficient water to cover them for several hours so they'll be soft enough to blend. Then simply drain off the water. Even those of us with high-speed blenders should take care to scrape down the sides and mix very thoroughly to achieve an ultra-smooth, non-grainy result.

Nutrition:

Calories: 295

Total fat: 14g

Cholesterol: 0mg

Carbohydrates: 38g

Fibre: 2g

Protein: 6g

Gooey Lemon Bars

Preparation time: 15 minutes

Cooking time: 25 minutes

Servings: 6

Bake: 347°F

Ingredients:

- For the crust:
- ¾ cup whole-wheat pastry flour
- 2 tbsp.Coconut sugar
- ¼ cup refined coconut oil, melted
- For the filling:
- ½ cup of organic sugar
- One packed tbsp. lemon zest (see Cooking Tip)
- ¼ cup fresh lemon juice
- 1/8 tsp. of sea salt
- ¼ cup unsweetened, plain applesauce
- 1¾ tsp. arrowroot (or cornstarch)
- ¾ tsp.of baking powder
- Cooking oil spray it can be(sunflower, safflower, or refined coconut)

Directions:

To make the crust:

In a small bowl, stir the flour, Coconut sugar, and oil together until well combined. Place in the refrigerator.

To make the filling:

In a medium bowl, add the sugar, lemon zest and juice, salt, applesauce, arrowroot, and baking powder. Stir well.

To assemble the bars:

Spray a 6-inch round, 2-inch deep baking pan lightly with oil. Remove the crust mixture from the fridge and gently press it into the pan's bottom to form a crust. Place inside the air fryer and bake for 5 minutes, or until it becomes slightly firm to the touch.

Over the crust, scrape and spread the lemon filling. Bake for about 18 to 20 minutes or until golden brown on top. Remove and leave to cool in the refrigerator for an hour or more. Cut into pieces until firm and cooled, and serve. To get each piece out, you could use a fork, as the pan is a little small for typical spatulas.

Cooking Tip: Don't let the idea of zesting a lemon scare you away if it's new to you! All you'll need is a fine grater or Microplane. The most important thing to remember is to gently zest only the yellow outer peel of the lemon because if you zest the white parts beneath that, it will taste bitter—and you're going for tart, not bitter. This tip applies to zesting limes and oranges as well, and once you get the hang of it, you'll find citrus zest adds a pop of flavour to a wide range of dishes!

Nutrition:

Calories: 202

Total fat: 9g

Cholesterol: 0mg

Carbohydrates: 30g

Fiber: 2g

Protein: 1g

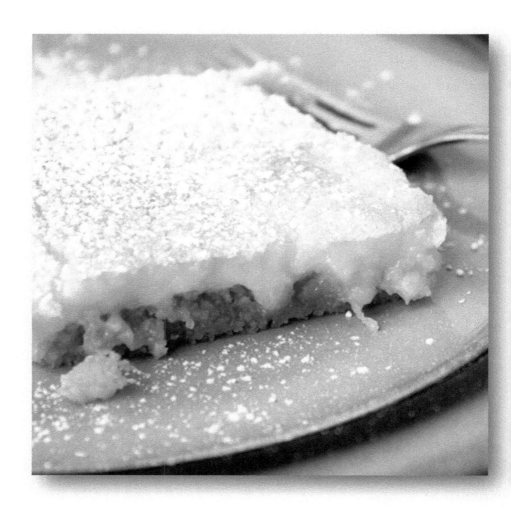

Raspberry Lemon Streusel Cake

Preparation time: 15 minutes

Cooking time: 45 minutes

Servings: 6

Bake: 311°F

Ingredients:

- For the streusel topping:
- 2 tbsps. organic sugar
- 2 tbsps. neutral-flavoured oil (sunflower, safflower, or refined coconut)
- ¼ cup plus 2 tbsps. whole-wheat pastry flour (or gluten-free all-purpose flour)
- For the cake:
- 1 cup whole-wheat pastry flour
- ½ cup of organic sugar
- One tsp. baking powder
- 1 tbsp. lemon zest
- ¼ tsp. sea salt
- ¾ cup plus 2 tbsps unsweetened nondairy milk (plain or vanilla)
- 2 tbsps. neutral-flavoured oil (sunflower, safflower, or refined coconut)
- 1 tsp. vanilla
- 1 cup fresh raspberries

- Cooking oil spray it can be (sunflower, safflower, or refined coconut)
- For the icing:
- ½ cup Coconut sugar
- 1 tbsp. fresh lemon juice
- ½ tsp. lemon zest
- ½ tsp. vanilla
- 1/8 tsp. sea salt

Directions:

To make the streusel:

In a small bowl, stir together the sugar, oil, and flour and place in the refrigerator (this will help it firm up and be more crumbly later).

To make the cake:

In a medium bowl, place the flour, sugar, baking powder, zest, and salt. Stir very well, preferably with a wire whisk. Add the milk, oil, and vanilla. Stir using a rubber spatula or spoon, just until thoroughly combined. Gently stir in the raspberries.

Preheat the air fryer for 3 minutes. Spray or coat the insides of a 6-inch round, 2-inch deep baking pan with oil and pour the batter into the pan .

Remove the streusel from the fridge and crumble it over the top of the cake batter. Carefully place the cake in the air fryer and bake for 45 minutes, or if a knife inserted in the center comes out clean (the top should be golden-brown).

To make the icing:

In a prepared small bowl, stir together the coconut sugar, lemon juice and zest, vanilla, and salt. If the cake has cooled for about 5 minutes, slice into four pieces and drizzle each with icing. Serve warm if possible. If you have leftovers, it can keep in an airtight container in the fridge for several days.

Nutrition:

Calories: 296

Total fat: 11g

Cholesterol: 0mg

Carbohydrates: 49g

Fibre: 4g

Protein: 3g

Pineapple Upside-Down Cake

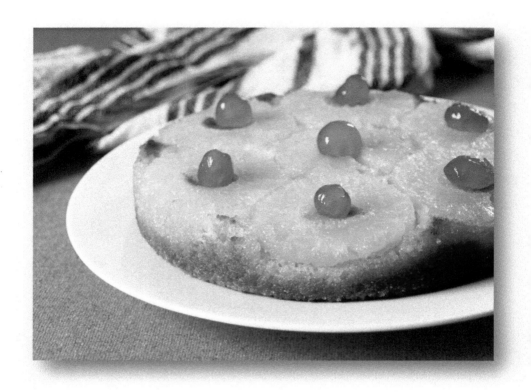

Preparation time: 10 minutes

Cooking time: 30 minutes

Servings: 6

Bake: 320°F

Ingredients:

- 1 cup whole-wheat pastry flour
- 1½ tbsp. ground flaxseed

- ½ tsp. Plus 1/8 tsp. baking soda
- ¼ tsp. sea salt
- ½ cup pineapple juice, fresh or canned
- 2 tbsp. melted coconut oil (plus more for greasing your pan)
- ¼ cup plus 2 tbsp. agave nectar
- ½ tbsp. fresh lemon juice
- 1 tsp. vanilla
- 1 to 2 tbsp. coconut sugar (for coating the pan)
- Three pineapple rings (fresh or canned)
- Creamy Lemon Sauce (optional)
- Vanilla or coconut vegan ice cream (optional)
- Vegan whipped topping (optional)

Directions:

In a medium bowl, add the flour, flax meal, baking soda, and salt. Whisk very well. Add the pineapple juice, oil, agave, lemon juice, and vanilla. Stir just until thoroughly combined.

Preheat your air fryer for 2 minutes. Gently grease the bottom and sides of a 6-inch round, 2-inch deep baking pan with coconut oil. Sprinkle to the bottom of the pan evenly with the coconut sugar (just enough to coat the bottom of your pan lightly).

Put the pineapple rings on top of the sugar in a single layer (you may need to break up some of the calls to do this). Pour the batter on top of the pineapple rings.

Carefully place the pan into your preheated air fryer. Bake and cook for 25 to 30 minutes, or until a knife inserted into the center comes out clean. Note: Your cake may look done before the center is cooked through, so the knife test is where it's at here.

Carefully remove the pan and allow to cool on a plate or wire rack for 3 to 5 minutes. Use a knife around the edges of the pan. Place a container on top (so that the dish is against the exposed cake). Gently flip over, so the cake is upside-down on the scale. Next, gently pull the baking pan off the cake so that the pineapple rings remain on top. Cut and serve—plain, or with Creamy Lemon Sauce, vegan ice cream, or whipped topping.

Nutrition:

Calories: 191

Total fat: 5g

Cholesterol: 0mg

Carbohydrates: 35g

Fibre: 4g

Protein: 2g

Blackberry Peach Cobbler

Preparation time: 10 minutes

Cooking time: 20 minutes

Servings: 4

Bake: 320°F

Ingredients:
- For the filling:
- 1½ cups chopped peaches (cut into ½-inch thick pieces)
- 1 (6-ounce) package of blackberries
- 2 tbsp. coconut sugar
- 2 tsp. arrowroot (or cornstarch)
- 1 tsp. lemon juic e
- For the topping:
- 2 tbsp. neutral-flavoured oil (sunflower, safflower, or refined coconut)
- 1 tbsp. maple syrup
- 1 tsp. vanilla
- ½ cup rolled oats
- 1/3 cup whole-wheat pastry flour
- 3 tbsp. coconut sugar
- 1 tsp. cinnamon
- ¼ tsp. nutmeg
- 1/8 tsp. sea salt

Directions:

To make the filling:

In a 6-inch round, 2-inch deep baking pan, place the peaches, blackberries, coconut sugar, arrowroot, and lemon juice. With a rubber spatula, stir well until thoroughly mixed. Set aside.

To make the topping:

In a separate bowl, combine the oil, maple syrup, and vanilla. Stir well. Add the oats, flour, coconut sugar, cinnamon, nutmeg, and salt. Stir well until thoroughly combined. Crumble evenly over the peach-blackberry filling.

Bake and cook for 20 minutes, or until the topping is crisp and lightly browned. Enjoy warm if at all possible, because it's beyond incredible that way!

Ingredient Tip: The sweetness level of peaches can vary so much! If you're using very ripe and sweet peaches, you may not need as much coconut sugar. You can also substitute frozen peaches here, as it's not always easy to find them fresh unless they're in season. One 10-ounce bag of frozen peaches is what you'll need for this recipe, but make sure to thaw and chop them before using them.

Nutrition:

Calories: 248

Total fat: 8g

Cholesterol: 0mg

Carbohydrates: 42g

Fibre: 6g

Protein: 3g

Vegan Snacks

Potato and Beans Dip

Preparation time: 10 minutes

Cooking time: 10 minutes

Servings: 10

Ingredients:

- 19 ounces canned garbanzo beans, drained
- 1 cup sweet potatoes, peeled and chopped
- ¼ cup sesame paste
- 2 tbsp. lemon juice
- 1 tbsp. olive oil
- Five garlic cloves, minced
- ½ tsp. cumin, ground
- 2 tbsp. water
- Salt and white pepper to the taste

Directions:

Put potatoes in your air fryer's basket, cook them at 360 degrees F for 10 minutes, cool them down, peel, put them in your food processor and pulse well.

Add sesame paste, garlic, beans, lemon juice, cumin, water, oil, salt and pepper, pulse again, divide into bowls and serve cold.

Enjoy!

Nutrition:
Calories 170
Fat 3g
Fiber 10g
Carbs 12g
Protein 11g

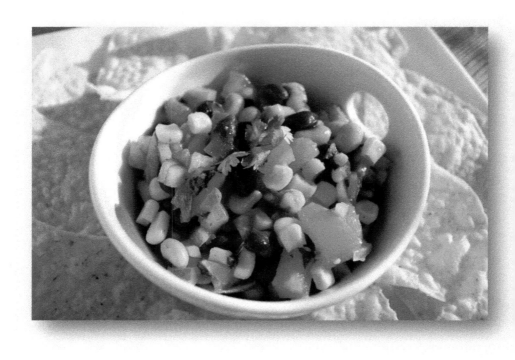

Cauliflower Crackers

Preparation time: 10 minutes

Cooking time: 25 minutes

Servings: 12

Ingredients:

- One big cauliflower head, florets separated and riced
- ½ cup cashew cheese, shredded
- 1 tbsp. flax meal mixed with 1 tbsp. water
- 1 tsp. Italian seasoning
- Salt and black pepper to the taste

Directions:

Spread cauliflower rice on a lined baking sheet that fits your air fryer. Introduce in the fryer and cook at 360 degrees F for 10 minutes.

Transfer cauliflower to a bowl, add salt, pepper, cashew cheese, flax meal and Italian seasoning, stir well, spread this into a rectangle pan that fits your air fryer, press well, introduce in the fryer and cook at 360 degrees F for 15 minutes more.

Cut into medium crackers and serve as a snack.

Enjoy!

Nutrition:

Calories 120

Fat 1g

Fiber 2g

Carbs 7g

Protein 3g

Basil Crackers

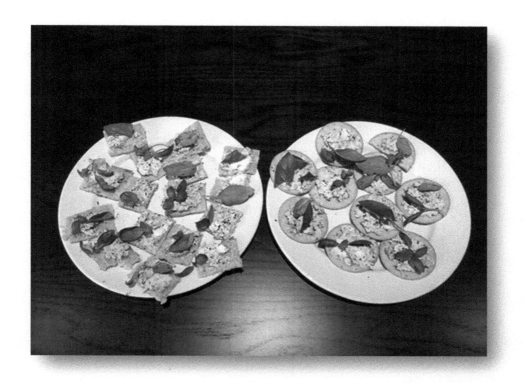

Preparation time: 10 minutes

Cooking time: 17 minutes

Servings: 6

Ingredients:

- ½ tsp. baking powder
- Salt and black pepper to the taste
- One and ¼ cups whole wheat flour
- ¼ tsp. basil, dried

- One garlic clove, minced
- 2 tbsp. vegan basil pesto
- 2 tbsp. olive oil

Directions:

In a prepared bowl, mix flour with salt, pepper, baking powder, garlic, cayenne, basil, pesto and oil, stir until you obtain a dough, spread this on a lined baking sheet that fits your air fryer, introduce in the fryer at 325 degrees F and bake for 17 minutes.

Leave aside to cool down, cut crackers and serve them as a snack.

Enjoy!

Nutrition:

Calories 170

Fat 20g

Fiber 1g

Carbs 6g

Protein 7g

Veggie Wontons

Preparation time: 10 minutes
Cooking time: 15 minutes
Servings: 10

Ingredients:

- Cooking spray
- ½ cup white onion, grated
- ½ cup mushrooms, chopped
- ½ cup carrot, grate d
- ¾ cup red pepper, chopped
- ¾ cup cabbage, grated
- 1 tbsp. chilli sauce
- 1 tsp. garlic powder
- Salt and pepper to taste
- 30 vegan wonton wrappers
- Water

Directions:

Spray oil in a pan.

Put the pan over medium heat and cook the onion, mushrooms, carrot, red pepper and cabbage until tender.

Stir in the chilli sauce, garlic powder, salt and pepper.

Let it cool for a few minutes.

Add a scoop of the mixture on top of the wrappers.

Fold and seal the corners using water.

Cook in the air fryer set the temperature at 320 degrees F for 7 minutes or until golden brown.

Nutrition:

Calories 290

Total Fat 1.5g

Sodium 593mg

Total Carbohydrate 58g

Protein 9.9g

Potassium 147mg

Vegan Bread and Pizza

Bread, Black Olives, Leek and Rosemary

Preparation time: 15 minutes

Cooking time: 30 minutes

Servings: 2

Ingredients:

- 4 tbsp. of wheat flour
- 1/3 of tbsp. baking powder
- 2 ½ tbsp. water
- 1 tbsp. olive oil
- Black olives
- One piece of leek
- Sesame seeds
- Rosemary to taste
- Salt to taste

Directions:

In a prepared bowl, mix all the dry Ingredients: 4 tbsp. of wheat flour, 1/3 of a tbsp. of baking powder, three pinches of rosemary and another two pinches of salt.

Mix well and add 1 tbsp. Of olive oil. Mix again. Add 2 tbsp. And half of the water and mixture also until you get a slightly sticky dough. Flour a clean table and put the ball of dough on top.

Knead well, can add more flour if necessary, to be able to knead with your hands without sticking.

Roll, make a churro and cut it into seven equal pieces. Shape each cut into a ball. Make a churro of each ball and flatten it with the roller.

Put the bread on the baking tray with the paper, and decorate them with black olives, finely chopped leek.

Bathe each bagel with ½ tbsp. Of oil, and add a pinch more of salt and the sesame seeds.

Bake at 4000F for 30 minutes and ready!

Nutrition:

Calories: 138

Carbohydrates: 22g

Fat: 3.7g

Protein: 3.6g

Sugar: 1.6g

Cholesterol: 0mg

Black Olive Bread and Rosemary in Olive Oil

Preparation time: 60 minutes

Cooking time: 40 minutes

Servings: 4

Ingredients:

- 1 lb. Wheat flour
- 1 cup of water
- 4 tsp. fresh yeast
- Pitted black olives
- Garlic powder
- Rosemary to taste
- Parsley to taste
- Olive oil
- Salt to taste

Directions:

Mix the flour with the 4 tsp. of fresh yeast, a tsp. of garlic powder, ½ of parsley, and two rosemary. Mix very well. Mix the yeast and spices with the flour that will give flavour to the black olive bread

Next, add 3 tbsps. of olive oil. Mix well, ensuring that there are a few lumps as possible. Add 1 cup of water.

With a shovel, mix all the Ingredients well and distribute the wet Ingredients among the dry ones.

Mix well until the dough acquires a manageable texture. Flour the table and smear your hands with more flour.

Remove the dough from the bowl and knead with force and energy for 8 minutes.

Now, shape and mold the dough into a ball and place it on a baking sheet and its greaseproof paper.

Stretch with a roller's help gives it an elongated shape, with rounded edges and a thickness of more or less 1 cm. Note that it will double in size, approximately. Let it rise for 1 hour. on the tray with the baking paper and covered with a cloth.

After the hour, paint the surface with generous olive oil so that the base is well greased.

On top, decorate with the sliced black olives, rosemary, salt and more garlic powder.

Now, put it in the air fryer at 3600F for about 40 minutes.

When it begins to toast, after about 30 minutes, if the bread is drying, you can repaint the top of the black olive bread with more olive oil.

Nutrition:

Calories: 138

Carbohydrates: 22g

Fat: 3.7g

Protein: 3.6g

Sugar: 1.6g

Cholesterol: 0mg

Homemade Chocolate Bread

Preparation time: 60 minutes

Cooking time: 40 minutes

Servings: 4

Ingredients:

- 1 lbs. Of flour
- 2 tsp. fresh yeast
- ¾ cup vegetable milk
- 1 bar of dark chocolate
- Orange peel
- Lemon peel
- 3 tbsp. of vegetable margarine
- Cinnamon powder
- A vanilla flavored soy yogurt
- Agave syrup or your favorite sweetener

Directions:

Put the flour in a large bowl.

Put the crumbled yeast with your hands. Beat with a fork until undo. Afterwards, cut a piece of orange peel and another lemon and let it marinate in the milk.

Add a minimum of ½ tsp. of cinnamon.

On the other hand, heat until the 3 tbsp. Of margarine is melted. When it is melted, add it to the flour and mix well. Add the yogurt, 2 tbsp. Of syrup and the flavoured vegetable milk, it has previously removed the lemon and orange peels and beaten with a fork to distribute the yeast well through the milk.

Knead well until the **Ingredients** are properly mixed.

Take the chocolate bar and chop it with a knife into small cubes. Add everything to the dough and knead for 3 minutes, with force and energy.

Sprinkle a little amount of flour on the table, put the dough on top, and knead for five more minutes.

Now, make a 'churro' and cut it into parts. Take each of the cuts, knead it and roll it.

Place the buns on the baking tray with the baking paper on. Let it rise for 1 hour. Afterwards, paint them with a little agave syrup, and with a spoon, spread it well over the entire surface of the bread.

Put in the air fryer at 360oF for 35-45 minutes. But check them after 35 minutes, try to be aware.

Nutrition:

Calories: 146

Carbohydrates: 2g

Fat: 5g

Protein: 2g

Sugar: 10g

Cholesterol: 0mg

Breakfast Berry Pizza

Preparation time: 7 minutes

Cooking time: 15 minutes

Servings: 6

Ingredients:

- 1 sheet of frozen puff pastry
- 1 Container of Vegan Strawberry Cream
- 6 Oz of fresh raspberries
- 6 Oz of fresh blueberries
- 6 Oz of fresh blackberries
- 8 Oz of fresh strawberries
- ½ Tsp. of vanilla bean paste
- ¼ Tsp. of almond extract
- 2 Tsp. of maple syrup

Directions:

Preheat your air fryer to about 390° F

Thaw 1 of your pastry sheets according to the Directions on the pack

Cut your pastry into its half and make fine cuts, with a knife, right on the top of each of the pastry sheet or poke it with a toothpick

Repeat the same process with the remaining quantity of the pastry

Put the pastry sheet in a greased baking tray and put it in the basket if the air fryer; then close the lid

Set the timer set to 15 minutes and the temperature to 390° F

When the timer beeps; remove the pastries from the air fryer and set them aside to cool for 10 minutes; meanwhile, prepare the topping by mixing the Vegan Strawberry Cream into a large bowl

Add the raspberries and mash the strawberries; then mix it with the raspberries, the vanilla paste, the almond extract and the maple syrup. Stir the mixture very well and when your crust becomes cool, pour the mixture over it with a spatul a

Top with the berries and the fresh strawberries

Serve and enjoy your pizza!

Note:

Some people prefer making a salty breakfast while others instead prefer having a sweet breakfast and at the same time a healthy one. This sweet pizza will be the best choice you can ever make.

Nutrition:

Calories 247.8 calories

Fat 6.1 grams

Saturated Fats 2.1 gram

Total Carbs 21 grams

Protein 25.4 grams

Vegan Main Dishes

Lemon Lentils and Fried Onion

"Fried onions alone might send you off a bit. Why add some lentils to the mix? It'll make the flavours pop out even more!"

Preparation time: 10 minutes

Cooking time: 30 minutes

Servings: 4

Temperature: 392degreesF

Ingredients:
- 4 cups of water
- Cooking oil spray as needed
- One medium onion, peeled and cut into ¼ inch thick rings
- Salt as neede d
- ½ cup kale stems removed
- Three large garlic cloves, pressed
- 2 tbsp. fresh lemon juice
- 2 tsp. Nutritional yeast
- 1 tsp. salt
- 1 tsp. lemon zest
- ¾ tsp. fresh pepper

Directions:

Preheat your Air Fryer to 392 degrees F

Take a large-sized pot and bring lentils to boil over medium-high heat

Adjust the heat into low and simmer for 30 minutes, making sure to stir after every 5 minutes

Once they are cooked, take your Air Fryer basket and spray with cooking oil, add onion rings and sprinkle salt

Fry for 5 minutes, shaking basket and fry for 5 minutes more

Remove the basket and spray with oil. Cook for 5 minutes more until crispy and browned

Add kale to the lentils and stir, add sliced greens

Stir in garlic, lemon juice, yeast, salt, pepper, and stir well

Top with crispy onion rings and serve

Enjoy!

Nutrition:

Calories: 220

Fat: 1g

Carbohoydrates: 39g

Protein: 15g

The Daily Bean Dish

"A traditional bean dish made using your Air Fryer! A healthy protein-packed meal at its best!"

Preparation time: 5 minutes
Cooking time: 8 minutes
Servings: 4
Temperature: 392degreesF

Ingredients:

- One can (15 ounces) pinto beans, drained
- ¼ cup tomato sauce
- 2 tbsp. Nutritional yeast
- Two large garlic cloves, minced
- ½ tsp. dried oregano
- ½ tsp. cumin
- ¼ tsp. salt
- 1/8 tsp. ground black pepper
- Cooking oil spray as needed

Directions:

Preheat your Air Fryer to 392 degrees F

Take a medium bowl and add beans, tomato sauce, yeast, garlic, oregano, cumin, salt, pepper and mix well

Take your baking pan and add oil, pour bean mixture

Transfer to Air Fryer and bake for 4 minutes until cooked thoroughly with a slightly golden crust on top

Serve and enjoy!

Nutrition:

Calories: 284

Fat: 4g

Carbohoydrates: 47g

Protein: 20g

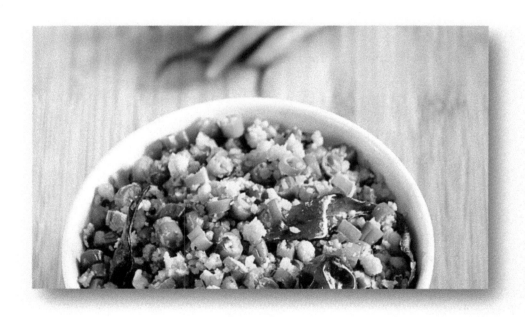

Fine 10 Minute Chimichanga

"If you are a fan of Deadpool, you've heard of chimichangas! This is your time to make a Vegan one!"

Preparation time: 2 minutes
Cooking time: 8 minutes
Servings: 4
Temperature: 392degreesF

Ingredients:
- One whole-grain tortilla
- ½ cup vegan refried beans
- ¼ cup grated vegan cheese
- Cooking oil spray as needed
- ½ cup fresh salsa
- 2 cups romaine lettuce, chopped
- Guacamole
- Chopped cilantro

Directions:
Preheat your Air Fryer to 392 degrees F
Lay tortilla on flat surface and place beans on center, top with cheese and wrap bottom up over filling, fold insides
Roll all up and enclose beans inside
Spray Air Fryer cooking basket with oil and place wrap inside the basket, fry for 5 minutes, spray on top and cook for 2-3 minutes mor e

Move to a plate and serve with salsa, lettuce, and guacamole
Enjoy!

Nutrition:

Calories: 317

Fat: 6g

Carbohoydrates: 55g

Protein: 13g

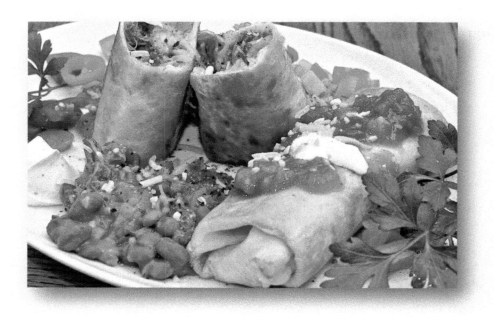

Mexican Stuffed Potatoes

"Stuff your Mexican potatoes style! You'll keep coming back to them, wanting for more!"

Preparation time: 15 minutes
Cooking time: 40 minutes
Servings: 4
Temperature: 392degreesF

Ingredients:

- Four large potatoes
- Cooking oil spray as needed
- One and ½ cups cashew cheese
- 1 cup black beans
- Two medium tomatoes, chopped
- One scallion, chopped
- 1/3 cup cilantro, chopped
- One jalapeno, sliced
- One avocado, diced
-

Directions:

Preheat your Air Fryer to 392 degrees F

Scrub potatoes and prick with a fork, spray outside with oil

Transfer to Air Fryer and bake for 30 minutes

Check potatoes at 30 minutes mark by poking them. If they are tender, they are ready. If not, cook for 10 minutes more

Once done, warm your cashew cheese and beans in separate pans

Once potatoes are cooked, cut them across top

Pry them open with a fork with just enough space to stuff the remaining Ingredients

Top each potato with cashew cheese, beans, tomatoes, scallions, cilantro, jalapeno, and avocado

Serve and enjoy!

Nutrition:

Calories: 420

Fat: 5g

Carbohoydrates: 80g

Protein: 15g

Vegan Staples

Tofu and Cauliflower Rice

Preparation time: 12 minutes

Cooking time: 20 minutes

Servings: 3-6

Ingredients:

- For round 1:
- 1 cup carrot, diced, around 1 1/2-2 carrots
- 1 tsp. turmeric
- 2 tbsp. soy sauce, reduced-sodium
- 1/2 block tofu, firm or extra firm
- 1/2 cup onion, diced
- For round 2:
- 1 and 1/2 tsp. of toasted sesame oil
- Two cloves garlic, minced
- 1 tbsp. ginger, minced
- 1 tbsp. rice vinegar
- 1/2 cup broccoli, finely chopped
- 1/2 cup of frozen peas
- 2 tbsp. soy sauce, reduced-sodium

- 3 cups cauliflower rice, OR cauliflower minced into smaller the pea-sized pieces

Directions:

Crumble the tofu putting the crumbled pieces into a large-sized bowl. Add the rest of the round 1 ingredient and toss to combine.

Put into the air fryer basket. Set the temperature to 370F and set the timer for 10 minutes – shake once halfway through cooking.

While the tofu is cooking, put all of the round 2 Ingredients in the same bowl to toss the tofu and toss to combine.

When the timer beeps after 10 minutes, add the round 2 Ingredients into the air fryer basket, gently shake the contents. Set the timer for 10 minutes, then shake the basket after 5 minutes.

When the timer beeps, check the cauliflower. If the cauliflower rice is not cooked at this point, then add 2 to 5 minutes to the Cooking time – shake and check every few minutes until done to your preference.

Nutrition:

Energy (calories): 119 kcal

Protein: 6.2 g

Fat: 5.72 g

Carbohydrates: 12.57 g

Roasted Carrots

Preparation time: 10 minutes

Cooking time: 25 minutes

Servings: 4

Ingredients:

- 1 tsp. herbs de Provence
- Two ounces or 4 tbsp. orange juice, about 1/2 medium-sized orange
- 2 tsp. olive oil
- 500 grams or 1 pound heritage carrots, or baby carrots

Directions:

Wash the carrots and slice into chunks; do not peel.

Toss the carrots with the oil and then toss with the dried herbs. Transfer to the air fryer basket.

Set the temperature to 180C and set the timer for 20 minutes.

When the timer beeps, transfer the carrots to the container you used to toss them with the oil and herbs. Add the orange juice and toss. Return the carrots to the air fryer basket. Set the timer for 5 minutes. Serve while still hot.

Notes: If using baby carrots, roast them whole – no need to slice into chunks.

Nutrition:

Energy (calories): 71 kcal

Protein: 1.05 g

Fat: 2.49 g

Carbohydrates: 11.91 g

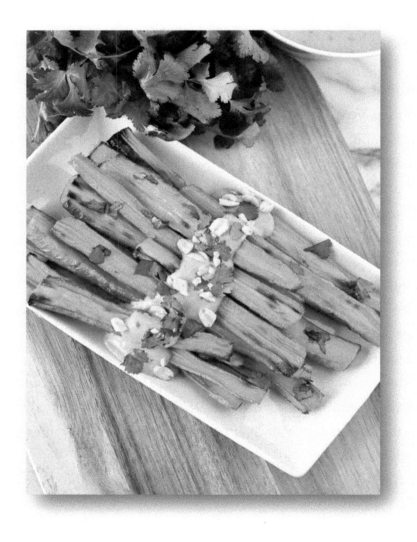

Lemony Green Beans

Preparation time: 10 minutes

Cooking time: 11 minutes

Servings: 4

Ingredients:

- One lemon
- 1 pound green beans washed and then destemmed
- 1/4 tsp. oil
- Black pepper, to taste
- Pinch salt
- Toasted nuts of choice, optional

Directions:

Except for the nuts, if using, toss the green beans with the rest of the Ingredients. Transfer to the air fryer basket.

Set the Air fryer's temperature to 400F and set the timer for 10 to 12 minutes.

Sprinkle with nuts, if preferred. Serve.

Nutrition:

Energy (calories): 47 kcal

Protein: 1.64 g

Fat: 0.56 g

Carbohydrates: 9.12 g

Roasted Rosemary Potatoes

Preparation time: 2 minutes
Cooking time: 10 minutes
Servings: 4

Ingredients:

- 1 tbsp. olive oil
- 1 tsp. rosemary
- Two potatoes, large-sized
- Salt and pepper

Directions:

Peel the potatoes and slice them into shapes for roasting. Toss with 1 tbsp. olive oil

Put those potatoes in the air fryer basket. Set the temperature for 180C and set the timer for 10 minutes.

When cooked, transfer to a serving bowl. Sprinkle with the rosemary and season to taste with pepper r and salt. Toss to mix well. Serve.

Notes: Do not overcrowd the air fryer – fill it half full at the most to perfectly roast the potatoes.

Nutrition:

Energy (calories): 177 kcal
Protein: 3.9 g
Fat: 3.59 g
Carbohydrates: 33.38 g

Scrambled Broccoli and Tofu

Preparation time: 5 minutes
Cooking time: 30minutes
Servings: 3

Ingredients:

- 4 cups broccoli florets
- One block tofu, chopped into 1-inch pieces
- 2 tbsp. soy sauce
- 2 1/2 cups red potato, chopped into 1-inch cubes, about 2 to 3 potatoes
- 1/2 tsp. onion powder
- 1/2 tsp. garlic powder
- 1/2 cup onion, chopped
- 1 tsp. turmeric
- 1 tbsp. olive oil
- 1 tbsp. olive oil

Directions:

Put the tofu in a prepared medium bowl and toss with the onion, garlic powder, onion powder, turmeric, olive oil, and soy sauce. Set aside and let marinate.

In a small-sized bowl, toss the potatoes with the remaining 1 tbsp.— olive oil. Transfer the potatoes to the air fryer basket. Set the air fryer's temperature to 400 degrees F and set the timer for 15 minutes – shake the basket about 7-8 minutes into the cooking.

When the 15 minutes are up, shake the basket again. Transfer the broccoli to a serving bowl .

Put the tofu, setting aside any marinade left in the bowl. Set the temperature to 370F and set the timer for 15 minutes.

Meanwhile, toss the broccoli with the reserved marinade. If there is not enough marinade, then add some soy sauce.

When there are only 5 minutes of **Cooking time** left for the tofu, return the broccoli to the air fryer and continue cooking for the remaining 5 minutes.

Nutrition:

Energy (calories): 446 kcal

Protein: 18.83 g

Fat: 17.38 g

Carbohydrates: 59 g

Whiskey Garlic Tofu with Veggie Quinoa

Whiskey Garlic Tofu with Veggie is a sticky, sweet and savoury favourite for any meal. Have it with a sandwich, salad or wrap.

Preparation time: 10 minutes
Cooking time: 10 minutes
Servings: 2

Ingredients:

- One block extra-firm tofu, pressed
- ¼ cup vegan coconut or maple sugar
- ¼ cup whiskey or bourbon
- 1 tbsp. apple cider vinegar
- Two garlic cloves, finely minced
- 1 tsp. onion powder
- Sea salt and black pepper, to taste

Directions:

If using an air fryer, line the basket with a round of baking parchment paper.

Once the tofu is pressed, slice it into half-inch slabs.

In a saucepan, combine the vegan sugar, whiskey or bourbon, garlic, vinegar and onion powder.

Stir continually, bringing to a boil, then reduce to a simmer. Simmer for about 10 minutes, stirring constantly.

Allow cooling.

Coat all the tofu slices and place them on a baking sheet lined with baking parchment paper.

Fry in the air fryer at 370 degrees Fahrenheit for 7 minutes.

Turn the tofu over and cook for another 3-4 minutes.

Serve over salad, mashed potatoes or with veggie quinoa.

Nutrition:

Energy (calories): 315 kcal

Protein: 23.98 g

Fat: 15.52 g

Carbohydrates: 25.32 g

Potato Fritter Sliders

Potato Fritter Sliders (Vada Pav) are an Indian snack food made in potato heaven! They are perfect served alongside sweet or savoury chutneys and sauces.

Preparation time: 15 minutes
Cooking time: 15 minutes
Servings: 3

Ingredients:
- For Potato Stuffing:
- Three potatoes, boiled
- 1 tbsp. canola oil
- Eight curry leaves
- ½ tsp. Black mustard seeds
- 1/8 tsp. asafetida
- Four cloves garlic, minced
- 1-inch piece ginger, minced
- One green Serrano chilli, minced
- ½ tsp. Salt
- ½ tsp. ground turmeric
- 2 tbsp. cilantro, finely chopped
- 1-2 tbsp. freshly squeezed lemon juice
- For the Batter:
- ¾ cup gram flour

- 1/3 cup water
- ½ tsp. Cayenne pepper or red chilli powder
- ½ tbsp. Oil
- ½ tsp. salt

Other Ingredients:
- Eight dinner rolls
- 2 tbsp. vegan butter
- 2 tbsp. tamarind chutney
- 2 tbsp. mint-cilantro dry chutney
- 2 tbsp. chilli-garlic dry chutney

Directions:

Mix all the batter Ingredients to form a thick and smooth paste.

Rest the batter while you prepare the stuffing .

For the Stuffing:

Mash the boiled potatoes using a potato masher.

In a pan on the stovetop, heat the oil. Add the mustard seeds and then curry leaves and let the mustard seeds pop.

Add asafetida, ginger, garlic and minced green chilli for 30 seconds until they are fragrant.

Add the salt, cilantro, turmeric, and potatoes. Mix well. Add the lemon juice and mix well.

Take the potato stuffing off the heat and set it aside to cool.

For the Potato Fritters:

Form medium-sized balls with the potato stuffing in the palms of your hands.

Brush the oil on the air fryer grilling pan.

Mix the batter, dip the potato balls into the batter, coat evenly, and place it onto the air fryer grill pan.

Cook at 390 degrees Fahrenheit in the air fryer for 14 minutes, checking halfway through cooking.

Remove the cakes from the grill pan.

For the Sliders:

Slice the dinner rolls into two pieces.

Heat the butter in a pan adjust over medium heat and place the sliced dinner rolls on the pan. Lightly toast the rolls and then apply tamarind and green chutney on both sides of the dinner rolls.

Sprinkle some chilli-garlic chutney on the rolls and place the patties in between the dinner rolls pressing gently.

Serve immediately.

Nutrition:

Energy (calories): 650 kcal

Protein: 15.15 g

Fat: 19.95 g

Carbohydrates: 106 g

Lightning Source UK Ltd.
Milton Keynes UK
UKHW020825170621
385666UK00005B/72